WHEN NATURE CALLS

Overcoming Shy Bladder Syndrome

Proven Strategies to Conquer Paruresis and Reclaim Your Confidence

ERIC LITTLE

ACKNOWLEDGEMENTS

First and foremost, I want to express my sincere gratitude to you, the reader, for choosing to go on this journey with me. Your support means the world and fuels my passion for writing.

This book would not have been possible without the encouragement and unwavering belief of my wife Sara. Her support, both emotional and practical, has been invaluable.

I am also deeply grateful to Bert and John for their contributions to this project.

Finally, I want to acknowledge the months of research, reflection, and countless cups of coffee that went into the creation of this book.

I hope this book brings you positive and lasting change and also makes your life more enjoyable.

Thank you again for your support.

ABOUT THE AUTHOR

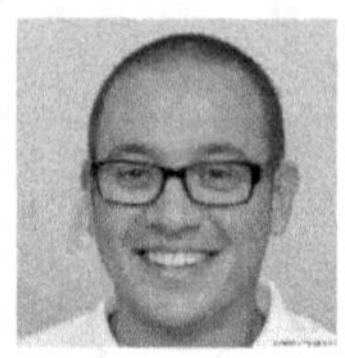

Eric Little is a globetrotting adventurer and a passionate advocate for personal growth. With a backpack on his shoulders and a curious mind, he has explored hidden gems across continents, from the bustling markets of Marrakech to the serene temples of Kyoto.

Eric's travel books are famous for being helpful and interesting. They not only tell you the practical stuff you need to know, but also give you a deeper understanding of the culture of the place you're visiting. He thinks that travel is more than just seeing sights – it's about meeting people, trying new things, and learning more about yourself.

When not exploring the globe, Eric dedicates his time to helping others unlock their full potential. His self-help books offer a blend of practical wisdom, inspiring stories, and actionable strategies for achieving personal and professional goals. He believes that everyone has the capacity for growth and that with the right mindset and tools, we can all live a life of purpose and fulfillment.

TABLE OF CONTENTS

INTRODUCTION

The first time I felt paralyzed in a public restroom, I was a teenager at a crowded stadium. The game was thrilling, the energy electric, but when halftime came, I found myself standing at a urinal, surrounded by a sea of noise and movement, unable to do the one thing I was there to do.

My heart raced, my palms grew clammy, and no matter how much I willed my body to cooperate, nothing happened. Eventually, I gave up and shuffled back to my seat, humiliated, my bladder still uncomfortably full.

I didn't know it then, but I was experiencing something called *paruresis*—also known as *shy bladder syndrome*.

At the time, I thought it was just because I was nervous. *"Just a bad day,"* I told myself. But the more it happened, the more I realized this wasn't a passing problem. It was showing up at airports, at work conferences, even during road trips when the rest stops were crowded. What baffled me was how simple it seemed for everyone else. How could something so basic—something I had done effortlessly my entire life—suddenly feel impossible?

If you've picked up this book, chances are you've felt something similar. Maybe it's the crowded restroom that sends your anxiety into overdrive. Or perhaps it's the fear of someone overhearing, or even the simple fact that others are present.

The situation may vary, but the feeling is universal: a sense of being trapped, of your own body betraying you in a moment when you just need it to function. It's frustrating, isolating, and often deeply embarrassing. But most of all, it feels like something no one else would understand.

That's the thing about paruresis, it thrives in silence.

For years, I didn't tell anyone what I was going through. I avoided situations where I might have to use the bathroom around others, making up excuses or meticulously planning my days to sidestep potential triggers. It felt like a secret I couldn't share, not even with close friends or family. After all, who would take me seriously? It's just going to the bathroom, right? But the more I hid, the worse it got.

It wasn't until I stumbled across a description of shy bladder syndrome online that everything clicked. For the first time, I had a name for what I was experiencing—and with that name came a strange, unexpected relief. I wasn't the only one going through this. In fact, millions of people struggle with paruresis to some degree, from mild discomfort to severe cases that disrupt their lives. It's more common than we realize, but because so few people talk about it, it's easy to feel like you're the only one.

That moment was a turning point, but it wasn't a cure. Recognizing the problem was one thing; figuring out how to overcome it was another.

I spent years learning about paruresis—what causes it, why it persists, and most importantly, what works to address it. It wasn't a quick fix, and it wasn't easy, but step by step, I found ways to take back control. And as I did, I began to feel something I hadn't felt in a long time: *freedom.*

This book is the guide I wish I'd had back when I was stuck in that crowded stadium bathroom, wondering what was wrong with me. It's not a magic solution, and it won't promise instant results. But it will give you the tools, insights, and strategies to understand paruresis and tackle it head-on. More importantly, it will remind you that you're not alone—and that this isn't something you have to endure forever.

Whether your experience with paruresis is mild or it feels like it's taken over your life, know that progress is possible. It's not about forcing yourself to "just get over it" but about approaching it with patience, compassion, and the right strategies.

You don't have to let this define you. With time and effort, you can reclaim the confidence and freedom you deserve.

Let's get started.

HOW TO USE THIS BOOK

This book was written with one person in mind: you; wherever you are right now on the spectrum of paruresis, however long you have been carrying this, and however much or little hope you are bringing to these pages. It was designed not merely to be read, but to be used: returned to, marked up, worked through, and kept close during the moments when you need it most.

Before you jump into Chapter 1, take a few minutes to read this section. It will help you get the most from everything that follows.

This Book Is for You, Wherever You Are

You do not need to have hit rock bottom to benefit from this book. You do not need to have a severe or long-standing case of paruresis. Whether your shy bladder is a mild inconvenience that occasionally frustrates you, or a condition that has quietly reshaped the boundaries of your entire life, the material here has been designed with your full range of experience in mind.

You also do not need to be ready to share this with anyone. No one needs to know you are reading it. Many of the most important early steps in recovery happen entirely in private: in the pages of a journal, in a quiet moment of honest self-reflection, in the small daily practice of a breathing technique that nobody around you even notices. You can begin exactly where you are, with exactly what you have.

How the Book Is Structured

When Nature Calls is organised as a progressive journey, each chapter building on the one before, taking you from understanding to action to long-term empowerment. Here is a brief map of the terrain:

Chapter 1 lays the foundation. It explains what paruresis is, how it works physiologically, and what it actually costs the people who live with it. If you have ever wondered whether your experience is real, clinically recognised, or shared by others, this chapter answers those questions clearly and compassionately.

Chapter 2 turns toward your personal experience. Using the concept of triggers; the specific situations, environments, and thought patterns that activate your paruresis; it introduces the trigger journal, one of the most valuable tools in this entire book.

Chapter 3 explores the cognitive dimension of recovery: how to identify the distorted thinking patterns that fuel anxiety, how to challenge and reframe them, and how mindfulness and *Acceptance and Commitment Therapy* (ACT) can transform your relationship with anxious thoughts from the inside out.

Chapter 4 introduces graduated exposure therapy, the cornerstone of effective paruresis treatment. It explains how and why the process works, and guides you step by step through building and using your own personalised fear hierarchy.

Chapter 5 gives you a practical toolkit of on-the-go techniques: breathing methods, progressive muscle relaxation, visualisation practices, and environmental strategies you can use in real situations, in real time.

Chapter 6 addresses the role of other people in your recovery, how and when to seek professional help, how to consider disclosure to loved ones, and how peer support communities can offer something that no book or therapist alone can fully provide.

Chapter 7 prepares you for the inevitable harder stretches, the setbacks, the difficult weeks, the moments when progress seems to have reversed. It offers tools for bouncing back, and makes the case for why celebrating progress is not self-indulgence but neurological necessity.

Chapter 8 brings everything together into a vision of long-term confidence and empowerment, not just freedom from paruresis, but the richer, larger life that becomes available when this condition no longer defines the boundaries of what you are willing to do.

How to Read It

For most readers, reading from beginning to end is the recommended approach, at least on a first pass. The book has been carefully sequenced so that each chapter prepares you for what follows. The cognitive tools in Chapter 3 make the exposure work in Chapter 4 more effective. The trigger journal in Chapter 2 informs the fear hierarchy in Chapter 4. The foundations are essential.

That said, this is your book and your recovery. If a particular chapter calls to you urgently, if you are in the middle of a difficult period and Chapter 7 on setbacks is what you need right now, go there. The book will still be here to read in sequence when you are ready.

Read with a pen in hand. This is not a book meant to be kept pristine. Write in the margins. Underline the sentences that land. Put a star next to the exercises you want to return to. Dog-ear the pages that feel most relevant to your experience. A marked-up, well-used copy of this book is a sign of genuine engagement, and genuine engagement is where recovery begins.

Do not rush. Some chapters may ask more of you than others. Chapter 2's trigger journal takes time to build. The fear hierarchy in Chapter 4 deserves real thought and honesty. Give yourself permission to sit with a chapter for a week before moving forward, if that is what the work requires. This is not a race, and there is no schedule to keep.

The Exercises and Reflection Prompts

Throughout each chapter you will find three types of interactive elements, each marked clearly:

Try This — practical, concrete techniques and exercises you can begin using immediately. Some are designed for quiet private moments; others can be deployed discreetly in the middle of a challenging real-world situation. Approach these as experiments rather than tests. Not every tool will work equally well for every person, your job is to find the ones that work for you.

Did You Know — research-grounded insights that explain why something works, or that offer a perspective-shifting fact about paruresis and anxiety.

Understanding the science behind your experience is itself therapeutic, it transforms bewildering symptoms into logical, explainable responses that can be addressed.

A Word of Encouragement — honest, warm reminders for the moments when the work feels hard, progress feels invisible, or discouragement is tempting. These are not empty reassurances. They are grounded in the reality that recovery from paruresis is genuinely achievable, and that the people who get there are not exceptional or unusually brave. They are people, like you, who simply kept going.

The Questions for Consideration at the end of each chapter are designed for journaling, reflection, or both. They are worth taking seriously. The quality of your engagement with these questions will significantly shape the quality of your progress.

A Note on Professional Support

This book is a self-help resource, not a substitute for professional care. For many people, particularly those with mild to moderate paruresis, the tools here will be sufficient to produce meaningful, lasting improvement. For others, particularly those with severe paruresis, co-occurring depression, or trauma at the roots of their condition, this book will be most powerful as a companion to professional therapeutic support rather than a replacement for it.

Chapter 6 discusses in detail how to find a therapist experienced in anxiety disorders and paruresis, and what to look for when you do. If at any point while working through this material you feel that you need more support than a book can provide, please seek it. Asking for help is not a sign that the self-help approach has failed, it is a sign of self-awareness, and it is one of the wisest things you can do.

One Final Note Before You Begin

The introduction to this book told Eric's story: the stadium at halftime, the years of silence, the slow and hard-won road to freedom. That story is real, and it is also, in its essential shape, the story of millions of people who have found their way through paruresis to a life that is genuinely, measurably larger on the other side.

Your story is not over. In fact, the most important chapters of it, the ones where you stop managing a limitation and start reclaiming a life, may be about to begin.

Turn the page. Let's get to work.

CHAPTER 1: UNDERSTANDING PARURESIS
You Are Not Alone, And You Are Not Broken

There is a moment many people with paruresis know intimately. You are standing in a public restroom; maybe at work, at a concert, or in an airport; and nothing happens. Your body, which moments ago felt urgent and ready, has suddenly gone quiet. You wait. You breathe. You listen to the sounds around you, hyper-aware of every footstep, every flush, every presence near you. Still nothing. A familiar wave of frustration, embarrassment, and helplessness washes over you. You leave without relief, telling yourself, again, that something must be deeply wrong with you.

Here is what we want you to know, right from the very first page of this book: nothing is wrong with you. What you are experiencing has a name, a well-understood mechanism, and, most importantly, proven paths to recovery. You are holding one of them in your hands right now.

What Is Paruresis? Defining Shy Bladder Syndrome

Paruresis (pronounced pah-roo-REE-sis) is a form of social anxiety disorder in which a person finds it difficult or impossible to urinate in the real or perceived presence of other people. Commonly called "*shy bladder syndrome*," it affects an estimated 7% of the general population, roughly one in fourteen people, making it far more common than most people realize. Yet because of the deeply private nature of the condition, it remains one of the most underreported and underdiagnosed anxiety-related conditions in the world.

Paruresis exists on a spectrum. For some people, it means mild hesitancy when using a busy public restroom, resolved with a brief wait. For others, it means being unable to urinate anywhere outside their own home, sometimes not even in a family member's house. In its most severe form, paruresis can make employment difficult (particularly in jobs requiring witnessed urine drug testing), restrict travel, strain relationships, and profoundly shrink the boundaries of a person's life.

It is formally recognized in the **Diagnostic and Statistical Manual of Mental Disorders** (DSM-5) under the category of **Social Anxiety Disorder** (Specific), and has been studied and treated by psychologists and urologists for decades. This is not a quirk, a weakness, or an overreaction. It is a genuine, diagnosable condition, and it responds well to treatment.

Did You Know?

The International Paruresis Association (IPA) estimates that as many as 21 million people in the United States alone experience some degree of shy bladder syndrome. Many have never told a single person.

The Science Behind the Struggle

To understand why paruresis happens, it helps to understand a little about how urination actually works, because this is not simply a matter of willpower or relaxation. Your bladder is controlled by an intricate two-part nervous system: the *sympathetic nervous system* (your "fight-or-flight" system) and the *parasympathetic nervous system* (your "rest-and-digest" system).

Urination requires the parasympathetic nervous system to be in charge. When you are relaxed, your brain sends a signal that allows the detrusor muscle, the muscle surrounding your bladder, to contract, while simultaneously relaxing the external urinary sphincter. The result is the comfortable, natural release most people take for granted.

Now introduce anxiety. The moment your brain perceives a social threat; being observed, judged, or embarrassed; the sympathetic nervous system fires up. Stress hormones like adrenaline flood your body. Your muscles tighten. Your focus narrows. And critically, the sphincter muscle at the base of your bladder contracts and refuses to release. This is not a conscious decision. It is your nervous system doing exactly what it was designed to do: protect you from perceived danger.

The cruel irony of paruresis is that the harder you try to urinate, the more anxious you become, the more your sympathetic nervous system dominates, and the tighter that sphincter holds. Effort becomes the enemy of relief. This is why people with paruresis often describe feeling like they are "blocked" or "frozen," even when their bladder is genuinely full and the urge is real.

This physiological response is not imagined and not voluntary. Brain imaging research has shown that people with social anxiety disorder demonstrate heightened activation in the *amygdala*, the brain's alarm center, in response to perceived social evaluation.

In people with paruresis, this alarm extends directly to the act of urination in social contexts. The body is reacting to a perceived threat as real as any physical danger.

Next time you feel the freeze of paruresis coming on, pause and notice, without judgment, exactly where you feel tension in your body. Is it your shoulders? Your abdomen? Your jaw?

Simply naming the physical sensation ("I notice tightness in my stomach") activates the prefrontal cortex and begins to quiet the amygdala's alarm. This is not a cure, but it is the first small step in learning to work with your nervous system rather than against it. We will build on this skill throughout the book.

The Hidden Impact of Paruresis

James, 34, is a project manager who travels frequently for work. He has managed his shy bladder for over a decade with an elaborate system of strategies: arriving at airports three hours early so he can use the single-occupancy restroom, booking hotel rooms far from the elevator so he is less likely to encounter people in the hallway, timing his fluid intake to the minute. He has never told his employer why he sometimes seems flustered. He has turned down two promotions that involved more travel. From the outside, James appears confident and capable. On the inside, he is exhausted.

Stories like James's are far more common than the silence around this condition would suggest. Paruresis is often described as an "invisible" condition — not because its effects are small, but because those who live with it become extraordinarily skilled at hiding it.

The practical consequences can be significant. People with moderate to severe paruresis may avoid or limit:

- Travel by plane, train, or long car journeys
- Attendance at concerts, sporting events, or cinemas
- Certain careers (healthcare, teaching, security, military service, jobs with drug testing requirements)
- Overnight stays away from home
- Romantic relationships and intimacy
- Social events involving alcohol (which increases the need to urinate)

Over time, these restrictions accumulate. A life shaped around a single anxiety is a life that quietly shrinks — not because the person is weak, but because constant management of an unspoken burden is deeply, genuinely tiring.

Emotional and Social Consequences

Beyond the practical, the emotional weight of paruresis can be heavy and complex. Shame is frequently at its center. Because urination is already a subject surrounded by social taboo, many people feel unable to seek help or even name what they are experiencing. They internalize the difficulty as personal failure, a flaw in their character or constitution, rather than recognizing it as a well-understood anxiety response.

Research has found that people with paruresis report significantly elevated levels of **shame, self-focused attention, and fear of negative evaluation** compared to the general population. These are the hallmarks of social anxiety, and they are treatable.

Depression frequently accompanies long-standing paruresis, not as an inherent feature of the condition, but as a consequence of sustained isolation, restricted living, and the grinding work of concealment.

Many people also experience anticipatory anxiety, a state of dreading situations before they happen, which can become as limiting as the paruresis itself.

The Vicious Cycle of Avoidance

Here is the most important thing to understand about how paruresis grows over time: *avoidance makes it worse.*

This is counterintuitive. When you avoid a situation that causes anxiety, you feel immediate relief. That relief feels like evidence that avoidance was the right strategy. But what avoidance actually does is send a powerful message to your brain: ***that situation was dangerous, and we were right to escape it.*** The amygdala records the lesson. The next time a similar situation arises, the alarm fires earlier, louder, and more insistently.

Over years, the circle of safe situations narrows. What once required only a quiet moment in a busy restroom may gradually require a private, locked, single-occupancy space. The condition does not stay the same when left unaddressed, it tends to expand to fill the space avoidance creates for it.

This is not a reason for despair. It is, in fact, profoundly encouraging, because it means the cycle runs in both directions. Just as avoidance teaches the brain that the world is dangerous, graduated, supported exposure teaches the brain that the world is safe. Healing is not just a matter of willpower or pushing through panic. It means gently, systematically providing your nervous system with new evidence.

That process; the science of it, the practice of it, and the real human stories within it; is exactly what the rest of this book is about.

A Word of Encouragement

If you have carried this in silence for years, or decades, it takes real courage to pick up a book like this one. You do not need to be ready to tell anyone. You do not need to have all the answers. You only need to be willing to take one small step at a time. That is enough. That has always been enough.

CHAPTER 2: FACING THE FEAR: DEMYSTIFYING TRIGGERS
Knowledge Is the Beginning of Freedom

There is something quietly powerful about the moment you stop asking "*What is wrong with me?*" and start asking "*What is happening to me, and why?*" That shift, from self-blame to curiosity, is one of the most important moves you can make on the road to recovery. And it begins here, in this chapter, with one foundational task: *understanding your triggers.*

A trigger is not a weakness. It is information. Every time paruresis flares in a particular situation, your nervous system is communicating something: **a learned association, a fear response, a memory encoded long ago as "dangerous."** Learning to read those signals, rather than simply dreading them, transforms you from a passive victim of anxiety into an active student of your own experience. And students, unlike victims, can learn their way forward.

Common Triggers and Their Roots

Paruresis does not manifest randomly. It clusters around specific situations, sensations, and thoughts that the brain has,through repeated experience, come to associate with threat. These associations vary from person to person, but research and clinical practice have identified broad categories that appear consistently across those living with shy bladder syndrome.

Understanding where triggers come from is as important as knowing what they are. Most paruresis triggers have their roots in one of two learning processes:

Classical conditioning occurs when a neutral situation becomes associated with anxiety through repeated pairing. The first time someone froze in a school restroom while being teased, the bathroom itself became linked to threat. Over time, the association generalized: any public restroom, any unfamiliar toilet, any situation resembling that original moment can activate the same alarm.

Cognitive appraisal refers to the meaning we assign to situations. If you believe that taking too long in a restroom means others will notice, judge, or mock you, then any situation where timing feels observable becomes a trigger. The actual danger is minimal, but the perceived danger is real enough to activate a full physiological stress response.

Both processes are normal features of human learning. And crucially, both can be unlearned.

Environmental Triggers

Environmental triggers are the external, situational conditions that tend to activate paruresis. They are often the most obvious, the ones people can name immediately when asked what situations they avoid.

Proximity of others is among the most universally reported triggers. Open-plan urinals with no dividers, restrooms where other people are audibly present, or even the sound of footsteps approaching the door can be enough to activate the freeze response. For some people, the trigger is direct proximity, someone standing at the next urinal. For others, it is merely potential proximity, the awareness that someone could enter at any moment.

Perceived observation or audience intensifies the response dramatically. Many people with paruresis find that stalls with gaps in the door, restrooms with poor locks, or situations where they feel somehow visible, even without being directly watched, create significantly more difficulty than fully private spaces.

Unfamiliar environments carry their own weight. A restroom at home, used hundreds of times, carries little threat. A restroom in a new city, a colleague's home, or a foreign country activates uncertainty on top of anxiety, making the already-difficult significantly harder.

Time pressure is a trigger that catches many people off guard. Ironically, needing to urinate quickly; before a meeting, between flights, at intermission; makes it less likely to happen.

The urgency generates its own anxiety, which activates the sympathetic nervous system, which tightens the sphincter further. Deadlines and bladders, it turns out, are poor companions.

Noise and silence can both be triggers, depending on the individual. Some people struggle most in very quiet restrooms where any sound they make feels amplified. Others find noisy, crowded restrooms overwhelming in a different way. The key point is that the acoustic environment matters, and understanding your particular sensitivity gives you valuable information.

Did You Know?

Research on social anxiety consistently shows that the anticipation of a triggering situation activates nearly as much anxiety as the situation itself. This means that much of the suffering associated with paruresis happens in the hours before an event; the morning of a long flight, the drive to a job interview; rather than only in the moment. Treating anticipatory anxiety is therefore just as important as addressing the situation directly.

Psychological Triggers

While environmental triggers are external, psychological triggers are the internal thoughts, beliefs, and mental states that fuel the anxiety response. They are often less visible, but no less powerful.

Meet Diane, 41, a secondary school teacher who has lived with moderate paruresis for most of her adult life. She can use restrooms that are completely empty without difficulty. But the moment a thought crosses her mind — **"What if someone comes in while I'm in here?"** — everything locks up. She has described it as a switch flipping. The restroom hasn't changed. Nobody has entered. Only the thought has shifted. And yet her body responds as though the threat were real and immediate.

Diane's experience illustrates one of the most important truths about anxiety: the brain does not reliably distinguish between imagined threat and real threat. The same physiological cascade; adrenaline, muscle tension, sphincter contraction; can be launched by a single anxious thought as by an actual event.

Common psychological triggers include:

Fear of negative evaluation — the belief that others are noticing, judging, or forming negative opinions based on how long you are in the restroom, whether they can hear you, or whether you exit without having clearly used the facilities.

Performance pressure — an internal demand to urinate on command, as though the body were a machine that should produce results when required. This pressure is self-generated, but it functions as powerfully as any external stressor.

Catastrophic thinking — the mental habit of imagining worst-case outcomes. "*I won't be able to go, I'll have to leave, everyone will notice, I'll embarrass myself completely.*" Each escalating thought feeds the anxiety that makes the feared outcome more likely.

Body hypervigilance — an intense, narrowed focus on physical sensations in the bladder and urethra, monitoring for signs of relaxation that never come precisely because they are being so closely watched. The act of observation itself disrupts the natural process.

When you notice a catastrophic thought beginning to build ("**What if I can't go and someone notices...**"), try naming it out loud or in writing: "**That's the anxiety talking**." You are not arguing with the thought or trying to force it away, simply labeling it creates a small but real psychological distance. Research in cognitive defusion (a technique from **Acceptance and Commitment Therapy**) shows that this labeling reduces the emotional impact of anxious thoughts without requiring you to believe they are false.

While the categories above are common, your experience of paruresis is uniquely yours. Two people with identical severity scores on a paruresis assessment may be triggered by entirely different situations: one by crowded airport restrooms, another by quiet office bathrooms. One by time pressure, another by perceived observation. Recovery works best when it is tailored to your specific pattern, which means the first step is learning what that pattern actually is.

This is where a trigger journal becomes one of your most valuable tools.

Keeping a Trigger Journal

A trigger journal is not a diary of suffering. It is a structured, curious, compassionate record of your experience, designed to reveal patterns that are difficult to see in the midst of a moment, but become clear over time when written down.

For each significant episode of paruresis difficulty (or successful navigation of a challenging situation), record the following:

The situation — Where were you? What type of restroom? What time of day?

Who was present (or could have been) — Were others in the restroom? Nearby? Was the potential for observation high or low?

Your anxiety level — Rate it from 0 (none) to 10 (maximum). This simple scale, used widely in CBT and exposure therapy, helps you track change over time.

Your thoughts — What was going through your mind immediately before and during the difficulty? Even fragments are useful.

Physical sensations — Where did you feel tension? What did your body do?

The outcome — Were you eventually able to urinate? Did you leave? How long did the episode last?

You do not need to record every restroom visit, only those that feel significant, difficult, or surprisingly easy. Aim for at least two weeks of consistent entries before reviewing.

Patterns and Insights

After two to three weeks of journaling, most people begin to notice something striking: their triggers are not random. Patterns emerge with quiet consistency.

You may discover that your anxiety spikes specifically in the late afternoon, when you are fatigued and your emotional resilience is lower. You may notice that your worst episodes cluster around performance contexts (before meetings, during social events) rather than ordinary daily routines. You may find that certain physical conditions — hunger, stress, dehydration — reliably lower your threshold.

These patterns are not discouraging. They are liberating. Every pattern you identify is a point of potential intervention; a place where a small, targeted change in behavior, environment, or thought can meaningfully reduce your burden.

One person reviewing their journal might realize: "***My worst moments are always when I'm rushing. If I give myself ten extra minutes before any situation where I might need to use a public restroom, my anxiety drops significantly.***" That single insight, drawn from their own data, becomes a strategy they can use immediately, long before any formal therapeutic work begins.

A Word of Encouragement

Looking honestly at your own anxiety patterns takes courage. There may be entries in your journal that are hard to write: moments that carry embarrassment, frustration, or grief for experiences you have missed. Please be gentle with yourself as you do this work. You are not cataloguing failures. You are mapping a terrain so that you can navigate it better. Every entry, however difficult, is an act of self-knowledge, and self-knowledge is where healing begins.

Before moving to the next chapter, take a few quiet minutes and write down your answers to these questions:

Which two or three situations are most reliably difficult for me?

What thought, if I'm honest, is most often present when paruresis is at its worst?

Is there a time of day, or an emotional state, when things feel slightly easier?

There are no right answers. Only your answers, and they matter enormously.

CHAPTER 3: COGNITIVE STRATEGIES TO REWIRE YOUR MIND

Changing What You Think Changes What Your Body Does

If you have ever stood in a restroom, completely unable to go, and thought **"*Just relax, why can't I just relax*?"** you already know that telling an anxious mind to calm down is a little like telling a fire alarm to stop being so dramatic. The alarm does not respond to instructions. It responds to evidence.

This chapter is about changing the evidence your brain receives, using specific, research-backed techniques that genuinely alter the way your nervous system processes threat. The strategies here draw from three of the most effective psychological frameworks for anxiety: ***Cognitive Behavioural Therapy*** (CBT), ***Mindfulness-Based Stress Reduction*** (MBSR), and ***Acceptance and Commitment Therapy*** (ACT). Each approaches the problem from a slightly different angle, and together they form a powerful toolkit for reshaping your relationship with paruresis from the inside out.

Challenging Negative Thoughts

The cognitive model of anxiety, the foundation of CBT, rests on a deceptively simple idea: it is not the situation itself that causes distress, but the meaning we assign to it. Two people can stand in the same busy airport restroom. One feels mild inconvenience. The other feels acute, paralysing shame. The restroom is identical. The difference lives entirely in the mind, in the rapid-fire thoughts and beliefs each person brings to the experience.

For people with paruresis, those thoughts tend to follow recognisable patterns. They arrive quickly, feel completely true, and carry enormous emotional weight. CBT calls them automatic negative thoughts, and the first step to dismantling their power is simply learning to see them clearly.

Identifying Cognitive Distortions

Cognitive distortions are systematic errors in thinking, ways the anxious mind bends reality to confirm its fears. Several distortions appear with striking regularity in paruresis:

Mind reading — assuming you know what others are thinking. ***"Everyone in this restroom knows I've been in here too long and they're judging me."*** The truth is that most people in public restrooms are focused entirely on their own business, their phones, or their own discomfort. The imagined audience is far more attentive and critical than the real one.

Catastrophising — predicting the worst possible outcome and treating it as certain. ***"If I can't go, I'll have to leave, I'll miss the whole event, and this will ruin everything."*** Catastrophising takes a genuinely uncomfortable moment and inflates it into a catastrophe, triggering a level of anxiety wildly disproportionate to the actual stakes.

All-or-nothing thinking — evaluating situations in absolute terms, with no middle ground. ***"Either I go normally, or I've completely failed."*** This binary framing leaves no room for partial success, gradual progress, or the reality that most situations fall somewhere in the messy, manageable middle.

Emotional reasoning — treating feelings as facts. ***"I feel like everyone is watching me; therefore, everyone is watching me."*** Anxiety is highly convincing. It generates feelings that are utterly real, but feelings are not evidence of external reality.

Fortune telling — assuming future failure based on past difficulty. ***"I won't be able to go. I never can in places like this."*** Each new situation is approached already defeated, before a single moment has passed.

Did You Know?

Research by cognitive psychologists **Aaron Beck** and **Albert Ellis** — the founders of CBT — demonstrated that identifying and labelling cognitive distortions reduces their emotional impact even before any behavioural change occurs. Simply naming a distortion ("That's catastrophising") activates the brain's rational prefrontal cortex and begins to dampen the amygdala's alarm response.

Reframing Techniques

Once you can identify a distorted thought, the next step is not to argue with it aggressively or replace it with forced positivity. That approach tends to backfire, the anxious mind is excellent at debating, and "*Everything will be fine!*" rarely convinces a nervous system on high alert. Instead, CBT uses a more subtle and effective strategy: *guided questioning*, sometimes called *Socratic questioning*, to gently expose the thought to scrutiny.

When a negative automatic thought arises, try asking yourself:

- What is the actual evidence for this thought, and what is the evidence against it?
- If a close friend told me they were thinking this, what would I say to them?
- What is the most realistic outcome here, rather than the worst possible one?
- Even if the difficult thing happened, even if I had to leave without going, could I cope with that?

That final question is particularly important. A great deal of paruresis anxiety rests on an unexamined belief that a difficult outcome would be unbearable, catastrophic beyond recovery. When you sit with the question honestly, the answer is almost always: yes, I could cope. It would be uncomfortable. It would not destroy me.

Consider Marcus, 29, a graduate student who had avoided using the restrooms at his university library for three years, instead making a fifteen-minute walk to a single-occupancy facility across campus. In therapy, his automatic thought was identified as: **"If I try and can't go, someone will hear, tell others, and I'll be humiliated permanently."** Working with a therapist, Marcus examined the evidence: Had he ever actually seen anyone mocked for spending time in a restroom? What was the realistic probability that a stranger would both notice and broadcast his experience? And if the worst happened, if he did feel embarrassed, what would that actually mean for his life?

Gradually, through honest examination, the catastrophe shrank to something closer to its actual size: an uncomfortable moment, not a life-defining disaster.

Keep a simple three-column record for one week. In the first column, write the triggering situation. In the second, write the automatic thought exactly as it appeared. In the third, write one alternative, more realistic thought — not a cheerful one, just a more accurate one.

Example:

Situation: *Busy work restroom before a meeting.*

Automatic thought: *"I won't be able to go and everyone will notice I was in there for nothing."*

Realistic alternative: *"Most people won't notice or care. Even if I can't go this time, I have managed difficult situations before."*

Over time, the gap between the automatic thought and the realistic one becomes easier and easier to find.

Practicing Mindfulness and Acceptance

Cognitive reframing works on the content of anxious thoughts, challenging what you are thinking. Mindfulness and acceptance-based approaches work on your relationship with those thoughts, changing how you respond to them, regardless of their content. Both approaches are valuable. Together, they are considerably more powerful than either alone.

Mindfulness-Based Stress Reduction (MBSR)

Developed by **Dr. Jon Kabat-Zinn** at the University of Massachusetts in the 1970s, MBSR is now one of the most extensively researched psychological interventions in existence. Its core practice is elegantly simple: paying deliberate, non-judgmental attention to present-moment experience.

For paruresis specifically, mindfulness targets two of the condition's most destructive features. The first is body *hypervigilance*, the anxious monitoring of physical sensations that paradoxically prevents the natural process from occurring. The second is *anticipatory anxiety*, the mental rehearsal of feared outcomes that begins long before any restroom is in sight.

Mindfulness practice teaches the nervous system a different response: rather than fighting sensations, narrating catastrophes, or desperately searching for signs of relaxation, you learn to simply observe what is happening with a quality of curious, unhurried attention. The breath is anchored. The present moment is the only thing being attended to. And in that quality of attention, the sympathetic nervous system very gradually quietens.

Research published in Psychiatry Research found that eight weeks of MBSR practice produced measurable reductions in anxiety severity and significant changes in amygdala reactivity, the very brain region at the center of paruresis. These were not just subjective reports of feeling calmer. They were visible changes in brain structure and function.

Try This: The 5-4-3-2-1 Grounding Practice

When anticipatory anxiety begins building; in the car on the way to an event, waiting in a queue; try this brief mindfulness anchor:

Name 5 things you can see. 4 things you can physically feel (the seat beneath you, the air on your skin). 3 things you can hear. 2 things you can smell. 1 thing you can taste.

This practice interrupts the brain's forward-projecting anxiety loop and returns attention to the present moment, the only moment, as it happens, where urination is actually possible.

Acceptance and Commitment Therapy (ACT)

Where CBT asks "*Is this thought accurate?*", ACT asks a different question entirely: "*Is responding to this thought in this way serving the life you want to live?*"

Developed by psychologist *Steven Hayes*, ACT does not try to eliminate anxious thoughts or feelings. It works from the premise that discomfort is an unavoidable feature of a meaningful life, and that the attempt to avoid or suppress anxiety often creates more suffering than the anxiety itself. *The goal of ACT is not to feel less fear. It is to act in accordance with your values even in the presence of fear.*

For paruresis, this reorientation is genuinely transformative. Instead of asking "*How do I make this anxiety go away so I can live my life?*", ACT asks: "*What would I do differently if I were willing to feel anxious and move forward anyway?*"

Three core ACT skills are particularly relevant.

Defusion — creating distance from thoughts by observing them rather than inhabiting them. Instead of "*I can't do this*," the defused version becomes: "*I notice I'm having the thought that I can't do this.*" That small grammatical shift creates real psychological space. The thought is no longer you, it is something you are observing, like a cloud passing through the sky of your awareness.

Values clarification — identifying what genuinely matters to you, independent of anxiety. *Do you value connection? Adventure? Professional achievement? Presence with people you love?* Paruresis costs you these things when avoidance becomes your primary strategy. Naming what you are actually fighting for, not just what you are fighting against, gives the work of recovery its deepest motivation.

Committed action — taking concrete steps aligned with your values, even when anxiety is present. Not reckless exposure, but purposeful, chosen movement toward the life you want, one small step at a time.

A Word of Encouragement

The techniques in this chapter are not quick fixes, they are skills. Like any skill, they feel clumsy at first, then gradually more natural, then eventually automatic. If your first thought record feels forced, or your first mindfulness attempt feels frustrating, that is not failure.

That is exactly what learning feels like at the beginning. Keep going. The research is unambiguous: these approaches work. And they work for people whose anxiety has been entrenched for decades, not just months. It is never too late to begin rewiring.

Reflection Prompt

Take a moment and write down your answers to these two questions:

What is the single most frequent negative thought that appears when paruresis is at its worst? Can you identify which cognitive distortion it represents?

What is one thing you have stopped doing — or never started — because of paruresis? What value does that thing connect to for you?

Your answers to these questions will form the foundation of the practical work ahead.

CHAPTER 4: GRADUAL EXPOSURE THERAPY — BUILDING CONFIDENCE STEP BY STEP

The Path Forward Is Paved with Small, Deliberate Steps

There is a moment in recovery that many people describe as a turning point, not a dramatic breakthrough, but something quieter and more surprising. It is the moment they realise that a situation they once dreaded has become... manageable. Not effortless, perhaps. Not entirely comfortable. But survivable. Even, occasionally, ordinary.

That moment does not arrive by accident. It is built — brick by brick, step by step — through a process called **graduated exposure therapy**. Of all the evidence-based approaches available for anxiety disorders, exposure therapy has the longest research history and one of the strongest track records. For paruresis specifically, it is widely considered the cornerstone of effective treatment. Understanding how it works, and how to begin applying it to your own life, is the subject of this chapter.

The Basics of Exposure Therapy
What Is Exposure Therapy?

Exposure therapy is a structured, systematic approach to anxiety treatment in which a person gradually and repeatedly confronts the situations, sensations, or thoughts they fear — in a controlled, supported way — until those situations lose their power to trigger a disproportionate fear response.

The theoretical foundation is a process called **extinction learning**. When you avoid a feared situation, the brain's threat-detection system (the amygdala) never receives the information it needs to update its assessment of that situation. Every avoidance confirms the implicit message: **that was dangerous, and we were right to flee**. Exposure therapy interrupts this cycle by providing the brain with new, repeated, corrective evidence: **I was in that situation. I felt anxious. And I survived. Nothing catastrophic occurred.**

With sufficient repetition, the amygdala gradually revises its threat rating downward, a process neuroscientists call **fear extinction.**

The situation does not disappear, but the nervous system's response to it changes fundamentally. What once triggered an overwhelming alarm begins to register as merely uncomfortable, then manageable, then eventually unremarkable.

For paruresis, this means systematically and gently approaching restroom situations that currently feel impossible, beginning with the easiest imaginable scenario and moving incrementally toward more challenging ones, only when you are ready.

It is important to say clearly: exposure therapy is not about forcing yourself into terrifying situations and white-knuckling your way through them. That approach, sometimes called *flooding*, is neither necessary nor kind, and for most people it is counterproductive. What works is patience, structure, and a deep respect for your own pace.

Did You Know?

A landmark study published in the **Journal of Anxiety Disorders** found that **graduated exposure therapy** for paruresis produced significant and lasting improvement in the majority of participants, with gains maintained at follow-up assessments months after treatment ended. Crucially, improvements were not just in restroom use, but in overall quality of life, social participation, and self-reported confidence.

Why Gradual Steps Matter

The word gradual is not a concession to timidity. It is a neurological necessity.

When anxiety is too intense; when a situation triggers an 8, 9, or 10 out of 10 on your anxiety scale; the brain's capacity for rational processing is significantly impaired. The **prefrontal cortex**, responsible for learning and updating beliefs, goes partially offline. The *amygdala* dominates. In this state, you are not learning that the situation is safe. You are simply enduring it, confirming once again that it is threatening.

Effective exposure works in the moderate anxiety range, roughly 4 to 6 out of 10 on your personal scale. At this level, anxiety is present and real, but manageable enough that new learning can occur. You experience the fear, remain in the situation, observe that nothing catastrophic happens, and the brain begins; slowly, incrementally; to revise its assessment.

That's why the order you choose is so important. You don't need to summon bravery to face your biggest fear right away. Instead, look for the perfect starting point, something that challenges you just enough without pushing you too far.

Consider Nina, 52, a hospital administrator who had managed moderate paruresis for over twenty years. She could use her home restroom freely, her private office restroom with mild difficulty, but any shared public facility was essentially inaccessible. Her fear hierarchy began not in a restroom at all, but with simply driving to a shopping centre and sitting in the car park, imagining using the facilities inside, until her anxiety dropped from a 5 to a 2. That was her step one. Three months later, she used a busy shopping centre restroom on a Saturday afternoon. She wept in the car on the way home, not from distress, but from relief.

Creating Your Personalised Exposure Plan
Developing a Fear Hierarchy

A fear hierarchy, sometimes called a SUDS ladder (*Subjective Units of Distress Scale*), is a personalised list of situations related to your paruresis, ranked from least to most anxiety-provoking. It is the map you will follow as you move through exposure work.

Building your hierarchy is itself a valuable exercise. It requires you to think concretely and specifically about your experience, not as a vague, global dread, but as a series of distinct situations with different anxiety ratings. This specificity is empowering. It converts an overwhelming fog into a set of addressable steps.

Here is how to construct yours:

Step 1: Brainstorm freely. Write down every situation related to urination and public restrooms that you currently avoid, manage with difficulty, or feel anxious even thinking about. Include imagined scenarios as well as real ones. Do not filter or judge, simply list.

Step 2: Rate each item. Assign each situation a distress rating from 0 (no anxiety) to 10 (maximum imaginable anxiety). Be honest. There are no right or wrong answers, only your authentic responses.

Step 3: Order the list. Arrange your items from lowest to highest rating. You now have a rough hierarchy.

Step 4: Fill the gaps. Look for large jumps in the ratings, for instance, a jump from a 3 to a 7 with nothing in between. These gaps need to be filled with intermediate steps, because jumps that large are too steep for effective learning. Can you imagine a situation that would rate a 4 or 5 and bridge that gap?

A sample hierarchy for moderate paruresis might look something like this:

Anxiety Rating	Situation
1-2	Using home restroom with a family member elsewhere in the house
2-3	Using a restroom in a trusted friend's home
3-4	Using a public single-occupancy restroom when no one is waiting
4-5	Using a public single-occupancy restroom with someone waiting outside
5-6	Using a multi-stall restroom when it is completely empty
6-7	Using a multi-stall restroom with one other person present
7-8	Using a multi-stall restroom in a moderately busy venue
8-9	Using a multi-stall restroom with no stall gaps and multiple people present
9-10	Using an open urinal or very busy, high-pressure public facility

Your hierarchy will look different, shaped by your specific triggers, living situation, and life demands. That is exactly as it should be. This is your map, drawn from your experience.

Set aside twenty minutes in a quiet, private space. Write freely, every situation you can think of, every scenario you have avoided or found difficult. Then rate and order them. You do not need to act on anything yet. The hierarchy itself is step one: a clear, honest picture of the terrain ahead.

Keep it somewhere private and return to it as your journey progresses, you will find, over time, that ratings you once wrote as 8s and 9s begin quietly to drop.

Practicing Exposure Safely

Once your hierarchy is built, the practice of exposure follows a consistent, repeatable structure that can be applied to each step-in turn.

Begin at the bottom. Start with your lowest-rated item, the one that produces only mild, manageable anxiety. This is not wasted time. Even small steps build the neural pathways of new learning, and early successes create momentum and confidence for harder ones ahead.

Enter the situation and stay. The critical principle of exposure is remaining in the situation until your anxiety naturally subsides, typically by at least 50% from its peak. Leaving at the height of anxiety reinforces avoidance. Staying, even without successfully urinating, teaches the brain that the situation is survivable.

The goal of early exposure sessions is not necessarily to urinate. It is to tolerate the situation with decreasing distress.

Use your cognitive tools. The reframing techniques and mindfulness practices from Chapters 3 and 4 are your companions here, not prerequisites. When catastrophic thoughts arise during exposure, practice gentle defusion: "***I notice I'm having the thought that this is unbearable.***" When body hypervigilance kicks in, try the 5-4-3-2-1 grounding practice to return to present-moment awareness.

Track your experience. After each exposure session, note your peak anxiety rating, how long it took to subside, and any thoughts or observations. This record serves two purposes: it provides data showing your genuine progress over time, and it builds a personal evidence base that directly challenges the catastrophic predictions your anxiety generates.

Move up the hierarchy slowly. Do not advance to the next step until the current one consistently produces only mild anxiety, a 2 or 3 out of 10. There is no schedule to keep, no timeline to meet. Recovery is not a race.

Moving too quickly risks overwhelming your nervous system and inadvertently reinforcing the fear response rather than extinguishing it.

Expect fluctuation. Progress in exposure therapy is rarely a straight line. There will be good days and harder days, steps forward and occasional steps back. A difficult session does not erase previous gains, the brain does not unlearn what it has learned.

A setback is information, not failure. It often points toward a gap in the hierarchy that needs an intermediate step, or a moment in life when your general anxiety and resilience are lower than usual.

A Word of Encouragement

The work of exposure is genuinely courageous. It is quiet and consistent and asks you to show up for yourself repeatedly, even when part of you would rather retreat. Every step you take on your hierarchy, however small, is an act of profound self-respect. You are choosing, deliberately and consciously, to reclaim territory that anxiety has taken from you.

Questions for Consideration

Before beginning your exposure work, it is worth sitting with the following questions. There are no right answers, only honest ones, and honest ones are the most useful.

Looking at my hierarchy, what is the single item I feel genuinely ready to begin with this week, not the most impressive step, but the most truthful one?

What support do I have available as I begin this work? Is there a trusted person who could know what I am doing, even if they are not directly involved?

What has avoidance cost me in the past year, in experiences missed, freedom restricted, energy spent managing and concealing? What might I gain by beginning to move in the other direction?

What would I tell a close friend who was doing exactly this work, who was nervous about beginning, unsure they could manage it? Can I offer myself the same words?

CHAPTER 5: PRACTICAL TECHNIQUES FOR ON-THE-GO RELIEF

Your Body Already Knows How to Do This, Let's Help It Remember

There is a particular kind of frustration that belongs uniquely to paruresis: standing in a restroom, knowing your body is physically capable of what you need it to do, and yet feeling utterly unable to make it happen. The knowledge that the mechanism works, that it has worked thousands of times before, makes the freeze feel even more bewildering.

But here is what that frustration is actually telling you: *the problem is not your body. Your bladder, your sphincter, your urinary system are all functioning exactly as designed. What has changed is the context, the signals your nervous system is receiving and the state it has entered in response.* And because the problem is in the nervous system's response rather than in any physical malfunction, the nervous system is precisely where effective intervention can happen.

This chapter is your toolkit, a collection of techniques you can use in real situations, in real time, to shift your body out of the *sympathetic* "threat" state and into the *parasympathetic* "safe" state where natural urination becomes possible. These are not tricks or hacks. They are evidence-based physiological interventions that work with your body's own architecture, not against it.

Breathing and Relaxation Methods
Diaphragmatic Breathing for Immediate Calm

Of all the tools available to regulate the nervous system rapidly, **diaphragmatic breathing**, also called *belly breathing* or *deep abdominal breathing*, has perhaps the strongest evidence base for immediate anxiety reduction. Its mechanism is direct and well understood: *slow, deep breathing activates the vagus nerve, the primary highway of the parasympathetic nervous system, which in turn signals the body to reduce heart rate, lower muscle tension, and shift out of the fight-or-flight state.*

For paruresis, this matters enormously. The external urinary sphincter, the muscle that locks during anxiety, is directly responsive to parasympathetic activation.

As the **vagus nerve** engages and the body shifts toward the rest-and-digest state, that muscle softens. You cannot force this relaxation through willpower. But you can invite it through breath.

Most of us, under stress, breathe from the chest; shallow, rapid breaths that actually signal to the brain that something is wrong, perpetuating the anxiety cycle. Diaphragmatic breathing reverses this completely. When the diaphragm drops and the abdomen expands on the inhale, the body receives an unmistakable message: *we are safe. We can relax.*

Try This: The 4-7-8 Breathing Technique

This breathing pattern, widely used in anxiety treatment and supported by research in autonomic nervous system regulation, is simple enough to practice anywhere:

Inhale slowly and quietly through your nose for 4 counts, letting your belly expand outward (your chest should move very little)

Hold the breath gently for 7 counts

Exhale slowly and completely through your mouth for 8 counts, as though fogging a mirror

Repeat this cycle 3 to 4 times. Most people notice a measurable drop in tension by the third repetition.

Practice this daily in non-anxious moments first, while sitting quietly, before sleep, or during a morning routine. Like any skill, it becomes more readily available under pressure when it has been rehearsed in calm.

A secondary breathing technique worth keeping in your toolkit is **extended exhale breathing**, *simply making your out-breath longer than your in-breath. A count of 4 in and 6 out, or 4 in and 8 out, achieves the same vagal activation without the breath-hold, which some people find uncomfortable.*

The principle is consistent: a longer exhale activates the parasympathetic system more strongly than the inhale. When in doubt, breathe out longer.

Did You Know?

Research published in the **Journal of Neurophysiology** demonstrated that controlled slow breathing at approximately 6 breath cycles per minute produced significant increases in **heart rate variability** (HRV), a direct measure of parasympathetic nervous system activity. Higher HRV is consistently associated with lower anxiety, better emotional regulation, and, critically for paruresis, reduced skeletal and smooth muscle tension throughout the body.

Progressive Muscle Relaxation

Progressive Muscle Relaxation (PMR) is a technique developed in the 1920s by physician **Edmund Jacobson** and refined extensively over the following century. Its core principle is elegantly simple: ***by deliberately tensing specific muscle groups and then releasing them, you teach your body to recognize, and deepen, the contrast between tension and relaxation***. Over time and with practice, this awareness allows you to release tension that you have been carrying unconsciously, often for years.

For paruresis, PMR addresses something critically important: the chronic background tension that many people carry in their pelvic floor, abdomen, and lower body, tension so habitual it has become invisible, yet which maintains a low-level sympathetic activation that makes urination consistently more difficult.

A full PMR session, practiced before bed or during a quiet period, works through the major muscle groups of the body systematically: feet, calves, thighs, abdomen, hands, arms, shoulders, neck, and face. ***Each group is tensed firmly for 5–7 seconds, then released completely for 20–30 seconds, with full attention given to the sensation of letting go.***

For on-the-go use in restroom situations, a targeted mini-PMR can be highly effective:

Try This: The Rapid Release Sequence

While standing or sitting privately in a restroom, work through this abbreviated sequence:

Shoulders: Lift them firmly toward your ears, hold 5 seconds, release completely. Let them drop as far as they will go.

Hands: Make tight fists, hold 5 seconds, release. Feel the warmth spread into your palms.

Abdomen: Draw your stomach muscles in firmly, hold 5 seconds, then let them go completely soft.

Thighs: Press your feet into the floor and tense your thigh muscles, hold 5 seconds, release.

Follow immediately with 3 cycles of 4-7-8 breathing. The combination of muscular release and vagal activation creates conditions meaningfully more conducive to natural urination than tension and controlled breath ever could.

Thomas, 44, a solicitor with severe paruresis, described his relationship with PMR this way: **"I had no idea how tense I was all the time. My shoulders were practically at my ears and I didn't even notice. Learning to feel the difference between tension and release, really feel it, was like discovering a switch I'd always had but never known about. I still use the rapid sequence every single time before I try a public restroom. It doesn't always work perfectly. But it always helps."**

Tools for Navigating Public Restrooms

Breathing and relaxation address the internal environment. But there are also practical, external strategies, grounded in behavioural and environmental psychology, that can meaningfully reduce the anxiety load before your nervous system even has to respond.

Creating a Sense of Privacy

For most people with paruresis, the perception of observation, real or imagined, is central to the freeze response. Anything that genuinely increases actual privacy, or that cognitively reduces the sense of being observed, directly addresses this core mechanism.

Choosing your environment strategically is not avoidance, it is intelligent scaffolding. During exposure work and in daily life, there is no virtue in choosing the most difficult possible situation when an easier one is available. Using a stall rather than a urinal, selecting a restroom at the end of a corridor rather than adjacent to a busy area, timing restroom visits during quieter periods, these are not crutches. They are sensible reductions of unnecessary difficulty, entirely consistent with gradual exposure principles.

Background noise is a consistently reported aid for people with paruresis, and its effectiveness has a clear rationale: sound masks the acoustic feedback that hypervigilance monitors so closely. Many people find that running the tap, using a white noise app on a phone (earbud in one ear), or simply choosing noisier environments reduces the acoustic anxiety load considerably. Some public restrooms have ambient music or hand dryer noise that serves this function naturally.

Occupying the mind, a technique sometimes called *cognitive distraction*, works by redirecting attentional resources away from body monitoring and toward an absorbing mental task.

Mental arithmetic (counting backwards from 300 in threes), reciting lyrics or poetry, planning a conversation, or mentally walking through a familiar route all serve to reduce the capacity available for hypervigilant self-observation. This is not using distraction as avoidance; it is interrupting the self-monitoring loop that sustains the freeze.

The phenomenon of **"observer effect"** in paruresis, where the mere belief that one might be observed is sufficient to trigger the freeze response, has been documented in research showing that even imagined audiences produce measurable physiological arousal equivalent to real ones. This confirms that privacy-enhancing strategies that work on perception as well as reality are entirely legitimate and effective tools.

The Power of Visualisation

Guided visualisation is a technique with robust evidence in both sports' psychology and anxiety treatment, and it is particularly well-suited to paruresis, where the problem exists substantially in the mind's interpretation of a situation.

Visualisation works by repeatedly activating the neural pathways associated with a successful experience, in the absence of the anxiety-provoking context. Over time, the brain builds a stronger, more accessible template for success, one that competes with, and gradually displaces, the well-worn template of failure and freeze.

A simple visualisation practice for paruresis involves finding a quiet moment; not in a restroom, but somewhere comfortable and private; and vividly imagining the following sequence in as much sensory detail as possible:

You approach a public restroom feeling calm and unhurried. You notice mild awareness of other people but feel grounded and present. You enter a stall, feel your body settle, breathe slowly, and feel the natural release occur easily and comfortably. You leave feeling relaxed and matter-of-fact about the whole experience.

The visualisation should be practiced daily for several weeks, always ending with the successful outcome. It should feel slightly idealized, more comfortable than current reality, because that is precisely its function: to build a neural blueprint for a future that does not yet consistently exist, but will.

Try This: Your Success Script

Write a short paragraph, 5 to 8 sentences, describing your ideal restroom experience in a situation that is currently challenging. Write it in the present tense, from the first person, including sensory details (what you see, hear, feel in your body). Read it slowly every morning for two weeks, pausing to genuinely imagine each detail.

Notice, over time, whether the scenario begins to feel incrementally more believable, because that sense of believability is evidence that new neural pathways are forming.

As you begin to explore and practice the techniques in this chapter, the following questions may help you reflect on where to start and how to build these tools into your daily life:

Of the breathing, relaxation, and visualisation techniques described, which one felt most immediately resonant, and which felt most unfamiliar? What might that tell you about where to begin?

When during your day could you realistically practice diaphragmatic breathing or PMR, not in a restroom situation, but as a daily maintenance practice that builds your baseline capacity for calm?

Are there one or two environmental adjustments; timing, location, background noise; that you could introduce this week to reduce the anxiety load of a situation you currently find difficult?

What would your Success Script say? Can you write it today, even if it feels aspirational, even if it feels far from your current experience?

The distance between where you are and what you write is not discouraging. It is the exact space that practice is designed to cross.

A Word of Encouragement

These techniques will not all work equally well for every person, or on every occasion. Some days the breathing will settle everything quickly. Other days it will take longer, or the visualisation will feel hollow, or the rapid release sequence will seem to do nothing at all. That variability is completely normal, anxiety is not consistent, and neither is recovery. What matters is that you keep returning to the toolkit, keep practicing in calm moments so the skills are available in harder ones, and keep meeting yourself with patience rather than demands. You are retraining a nervous system that has been protecting you for years in the only way it knew how. That takes time. And it is absolutely, completely worth it.

CHAPTER 6: LEVERAGING SUPPORT NETWORKS

You Were Never Meant to Carry This Alone

There is a particular loneliness that comes with paruresis. Not the loneliness of being physically isolated, most people with shy bladder syndrome have full lives, relationships, and social connections. It is a more specific kind: the loneliness of carrying something significant that nobody around you knows about. Of navigating a daily challenge that shapes your decisions, limits your freedom, and costs you energy, in complete silence.

For many people, that silence has lasted years. Decades, sometimes. And while the silence feels protective; avoiding the imagined horror of having to explain, of being misunderstood or dismissed or, worst of all, laughed at; it carries its own considerable cost. Because one of the most consistently replicated findings in anxiety research is this: social support is not merely comforting. It is therapeutically active. Connection with others; whether a trusted partner, a compassionate therapist, or a peer who genuinely understands; does not just make the journey more bearable. It measurably accelerates recovery.

This chapter is about opening that circle. Carefully, at your own pace, in the ways that feel right for you, but opening it nonetheless.

Seeking Professional Help
When to Consult a Therapist

Many people with paruresis manage for years without professional support; developing their own coping strategies, reading widely, and making incremental progress through self-directed effort. Self-help resources, including this book, can be genuinely effective, particularly for mild to moderate paruresis. There is no rule that says professional help is required before you can begin recovering.

That said, there are circumstances where working with a trained therapist is not just helpful but strongly advisable, and recognising those circumstances is itself an act of self-awareness and self-care.

Consider seeking professional support if:

Your paruresis is significantly restricting your life. If you are turning down job opportunities, avoiding travel, declining social invitations, or structuring your entire daily routine around restroom management, the condition has moved beyond a manageable inconvenience into territory where professional guidance will almost certainly accelerate your progress.

Self-directed exposure feels consistently overwhelming. Some people find that even the lowest steps on their fear hierarchy produce anxiety that is too intense to work with alone. A therapist provides real-time support, can help calibrate the pace of exposure, and offers a relational safety that makes the work more manageable.

Depression or significant shame accompanies the anxiety. As discussed in Chapter 1, paruresis frequently co-occurs with depression, particularly when it has been present for many years. If you notice persistent low mood, withdrawal from activities you once valued, or a pervasive sense of hopelessness about recovery, professional support is genuinely important, not because paruresis has made you mentally unwell, but because untreated depression makes every other form of therapeutic work harder.

You have experienced trauma connected to the condition. For some people, paruresis began following a specific humiliating or distressing incident: public teasing, a shaming experience in childhood, a witnessed episode of extreme embarrassment. Where trauma is present at the roots, trauma-informed therapeutic approaches may be needed before or alongside standard exposure work.

Did You Know?

Research consistently shows that the combination of self-help resources and professional therapeutic support produces better outcomes than either alone. If you have been working with this book and finding it helpful, adding even a small number of sessions with a trained anxiety therapist can meaningfully amplify your progress, not because the self-help work isn't working, but because the two approaches reinforce each other.

Effective Therapy Modalities

Not all therapy is equally effective for paruresis, and knowing what to look for when seeking help can save considerable time and frustration. The approaches with the strongest evidence base are the same frameworks introduced in Chapter 3, now applied within a therapeutic relationship:

Cognitive Behavioural Therapy (CBT) remains the most extensively researched treatment for social anxiety disorder, including paruresis. A CBT therapist will work systematically through the cognitive distortions maintaining your anxiety, help you build and navigate your exposure hierarchy, and provide structured skills development across the full range of techniques covered in this book. Look for a therapist with specific experience in anxiety disorders and, ideally, some familiarity with paruresis or social anxiety in its more specific presentations.

Acceptance and Commitment Therapy (ACT) is increasingly recognised as highly effective for paruresis, particularly for people who have found cognitive challenging alone to be insufficient. ACT's emphasis on values-based action, psychological flexibility, and defusion from anxious thoughts complements exposure work particularly well.

EMDR (**Eye Movement Desensitisation and Reprocessing**) may be relevant where paruresis has clear traumatic roots, a specific incident that is vividly remembered and continues to generate intense distress. EMDR works to reprocess the emotional charge attached to traumatic memories, reducing their power to activate the present-day anxiety response.

Group therapy deserves particular mention. For paruresis specifically, the experience of working through exposure exercises alongside others who share the same struggle carries a therapeutic potency that individual therapy sometimes cannot replicate.

The normalisation that comes from sitting in a room with ten other people who completely understand your experience; without explanation, without embarrassment; is itself a significant therapeutic event.

When approaching a new therapist, it is entirely reasonable to ask directly: "Do you have experience working with social anxiety disorder and specifically with paruresis or similar conditions?"

A good therapist will welcome this question. If a therapist dismisses the condition as trivial or responds with confusion about what paruresis is, that is useful information, and a good reason to seek someone else.

Try This: Preparing for Your First Therapy Appointment

Many people with paruresis find the prospect of explaining the condition to a therapist, the very first conversation, anxiety-provoking in its own right. It can help to write a brief, honest summary beforehand: when it began, how it affects your daily life, what you have already tried, and what you most hope to achieve through therapy.

You do not need to read this aloud, simply having it written prepares your thoughts and reduces the cognitive load of that first difficult disclosure. Some people email it to their therapist before the session, which can make the first meeting feel less like starting from scratch.

Building a Supportive Circle
Connecting with Loved Ones

The decision to tell someone close to you about your paruresis is deeply personal, and there is no universal right answer about whether, when, or how to do it. Some people find that disclosure, even to a single trusted person, produces an almost physical sense of relief, as though a weight has been lifted that they had grown so accustomed to they had stopped noticing its presence.

Others disclose and find the response underwhelming or clumsy, and feel temporarily worse. Both experiences are valid. Both, ultimately, are survivable.

What research on disclosure and social anxiety tells us is that the anticipation of negative response is almost always worse than the actual response. The imagined reaction; mockery, contempt, bewilderment, dismissal; is typically far more damaging than what actually occurs when someone who cares about you is told something important about your experience.

Priya, 38, a marketing director, described telling her husband of six years about her paruresis after hiding it for their entire relationship. **"I had this whole speech prepared. I was shaking. I genuinely thought he might think less of me, that it would change how he saw me."** His actual response, she reported, was to pause, nod thoughtfully, and say: **"So that's why you always seem stressed before long drives. I thought I'd done something wrong."** He had noticed something was difficult. He had drawn the wrong conclusion and blamed himself. Her disclosure did not introduce a problem into the relationship. It resolved one that had silently existed for years.

If and when you choose to tell someone, a few principles tend to make the conversation more productive:

Choose your person carefully. The first disclosure does not need to go to the most important person in your life. It can go to the person most likely to respond with warmth and without judgment; a sibling, a close friend, a partner who has already demonstrated their capacity for empathy in other contexts.

Frame it clearly. Paruresis is a recognised anxiety condition, not a personal quirk or a mystery. Naming it — ***"It's called paruresis. It's a form of social anxiety that affects about one in fourteen people"*** — immediately shifts the conversation from the territory of embarrassment into the territory of information. Most people respond more helpfully to something named and explained than to something vague and undefined.

Be specific about what you need. Do you want the person to simply know? To occasionally check in? To be a practice partner for exposure exercises? To stop commenting when you decline certain situations? Loved ones generally want to help but frequently do not know how. Giving them a specific, manageable role transforms good intentions into genuine support.

A Word of Encouragement

If the idea of telling anyone feels completely impossible right now, that is perfectly okay. You do not need to disclose to anyone to begin recovering. This chapter is about what becomes available to you when you are ready to open the circle, not a prescription for what you must do immediately.

Plant the seed. Let it sit. You may find, as you progress through the work of this book, that what once felt impossible gradually begins to feel merely difficult, and then possible, and then done.

Joining Peer Support Groups

There is something that professional therapy and personal relationships, however valuable, cannot fully provide: *the experience of being truly, specifically understood by someone who has lived what you have lived.*

Peer support groups for paruresis, both in-person and online, offer exactly this. ***The International Paruresis Association*** (IPA) facilitates workshops, telephone support groups, and an online community where people at every stage of recovery connect, share strategies, celebrate progress, and offer the kind of matter-of-fact, unsentimental encouragement that only comes from shared experience.

There is no need to explain what it feels like to time your fluid intake around a social event, or to feel the particular dread of a job that requires a witnessed drug test. In a paruresis peer community, these experiences are simply understood.

The therapeutic value of peer support is well-documented. Research on peer groups for anxiety and related conditions consistently finds that participants report reduced shame, increased motivation, greater persistence with therapeutic techniques, and meaningfully improved outcomes compared to those working entirely alone.

The mechanism is not mysterious: when you see someone further along the recovery path than you, someone who once couldn't use a restroom outside their home and now travels internationally, the brain's implicit belief that recovery is impossible for you specifically begins to shift. Evidence is evidence, wherever it comes from.

Online communities offer particular accessibility for people whose paruresis, geographic location, or schedule make in-person groups difficult. Forums, closed social media groups, and moderated discussion boards allow people to connect, ask questions, and share progress at whatever level of anonymity feels safe.

For many people, the first disclosure they ever make about paruresis is in an online community where nobody knows their name, and that anonymous first step turns out to be the one that changes everything.

Try This: Your First Step Toward Connection

This week, take one small step toward widening your support circle. This might mean:

Visiting the International Paruresis Association website and reading one account written by someone in recovery

Writing, even if you never send it, what you would want a trusted person to know about your experience

Searching for an online peer support group and reading (without posting, if that feels like enough for now) what others have shared

You do not need to leap into full disclosure or community participation. You only need to take one step toward the knowledge that you are not alone in this, because you are not. You never were.

Questions for Consideration

As you reflect on this chapter, consider sitting with the following questions at a pace that feels comfortable:

Is there one person in my life — just one — to whom I might, at some point, consider disclosing my paruresis? What would need to feel different before that conversation became possible?

Looking honestly at my current situation, are there signs that professional therapeutic support might meaningfully accelerate my progress, not because I am failing, but because I deserve more help than I am currently giving myself?

What has the silence cost me? Not in terms of restroom use, but in terms of intimacy, authenticity, and the energy spent on concealment? Is that a cost I want to keep paying?

What would it mean to me to be genuinely understood; by a therapist, a loved one, or a peer who shares this experience? Can I let myself want that?

CHAPTER 7: OVERCOMING SETBACKS AND STAYING MOTIVATED

Progress Is Rarely a Straight Line, And That Is Completely Normal

Picture the recovery journey as a mountain path rather than an escalator. An escalator moves in one direction only — smooth, mechanical, inevitable. A mountain path winds. It doubles back on itself sometimes. There are stretches where the gradient eases and the view opens up gloriously, and stretches where the path narrows, the weather closes in, and you wonder whether you have lost your way entirely. And then the path opens again.

Nobody who has climbed a mountain considers the switchbacks a failure. They are simply the nature of the terrain.

Recovery from paruresis follows the same geography. There will be weeks of genuine, heartening progress: situations navigated that once seemed impossible, anxiety ratings that have quietly dropped, moments of ordinary freedom that feel quietly extraordinary. And there will be harder periods: a difficult week at work that raises baseline anxiety across the board, a situation that triggers an unexpectedly strong response, a run of days where the tools feel less available and the old patterns reassert themselves with unwelcome familiarity.

Both are part of the same journey. This chapter is about how to navigate the harder stretches, not just surviving them, but extracting from them the information and resilience that will ultimately make you stronger.

Handling Relapses with Resilience
Normalising Setbacks

The single most important thing to understand about setbacks in anxiety recovery is this: they are not evidence that you are failing. They are evidence that you are human.

Anxiety treatment research is unambiguous on this point. Setbacks, periods of increased symptom severity following improvement, are a normal, expected, and well-documented feature of recovery from anxiety disorders, including paruresis. A landmark review of CBT outcomes published in **Clinical Psychology Review** found that temporary return of symptoms occurred in the majority of participants at some point during or after treatment, and crucially, that these setbacks did not predict long-term outcomes. What predicted outcomes was not the absence of setbacks, but the response to them.

This distinction is worth sitting with. The setback itself is not the problem. The interpretation of the setback, what you tell yourself it means, is where the real risk lies.

When a difficult period is interpreted as evidence of fundamental failure — *"I'm back to square one," "This will never work for me," "I've lost everything I worked for"* — the resulting discouragement frequently leads to reduced effort, increased avoidance, and a genuine worsening of symptoms. The interpretation becomes a self-fulfilling prophecy.

When the same difficult period is interpreted accurately — *"This is a temporary increase in symptoms, which is normal in recovery. It does not erase my progress. It is telling me something useful"* — the response is entirely different. Curiosity replaces despair. The person examines what has changed, adjusts their approach if necessary, and continues forward.

Did You Know?

Neuroscience research on fear extinction, the process underlying exposure therapy, has demonstrated that extinguished fear responses can temporarily return under three specific conditions: stress (when general life pressures are elevated), context change (when you encounter the feared situation in a new or unexpected setting), and time (after a period without practice).

Understanding these three triggers transforms a "relapse" from a mysterious failure into a predictable, explainable event, one that can be directly addressed.

Consider Oliver, 47, a secondary school teacher who had made substantial progress over eight months of self-directed exposure work. He had moved from being unable to use any facility outside his home to regularly using the staff restrooms at work and even the facilities at his local gym. Then his school underwent a major restructuring. For three months, he was under sustained professional pressure unlike anything he had experienced in years. His paruresis worsened noticeably. He found himself avoiding the gym again, and even the staff restroom felt difficult on bad days.

His first response was despair: **"Eight months of work gone. I'm back where I started."** His second response, arrived at after a difficult week and a conversation with a trusted friend, was more accurate: **"My baseline anxiety has risen significantly because of external stress, and that's affecting everything, including this. This isn't failure. This is my nervous system being overloaded. What do I need right now?"**

What Oliver needed was not to immediately resume his full exposure hierarchy, but to return to fundamentals: daily breathing practice, PMR, and the lower rungs of his hierarchy where success was reliably achievable. Within six weeks of the restructuring settling, his paruresis had returned to the level it had been before the stressful period, and he had learned something invaluable about the relationship between his general stress load and his symptoms.

Tools for Bouncing Back

When a setback occurs, having a structured response prevents the paralysis that despair creates. The following sequence offers a practical framework:

Step 1: Name it without judgment. Simply acknowledge what is happening: ***"I'm having a harder period right now."*** Not ***"I've failed"*** or ***"This is a disaster"*** — just an honest, neutral observation. The language you use in this moment matters more than it might seem.

Step 2: Look for the context. Has something changed in your life recently? Elevated stress at work or home? Disrupted sleep? Illness? A significant life transition? Setbacks rarely occur in a vacuum. Identifying the contributing context transforms the setback from a mysterious regression into a logical consequence, and logical consequences can be addressed.

Step 3: Return to your foundations. Before resuming exposure work at its current level, spend a week or two reinvesting in the foundational practices: daily diaphragmatic breathing, progressive muscle relaxation, mindfulness, and the cognitive tools from Chapter 3. Think of these as restoring your baseline capacity before asking your nervous system to stretch again.

Step 4: Step back on the hierarchy, temporarily. There is no shame in returning to a lower rung of your exposure ladder for a period. This is not retreat, it is intelligent recalibration. Rebuilding confidence at a manageable level reactivates the neural pathways of success and creates a secure platform from which to re-advance.

Step 5: Reconnect with your support. If you have a therapist, this is the moment to reach out. If you have a trusted person who knows about your journey, tell them you are having a harder period. If you have been engaging with a peer community, return to it. Isolation during setbacks feeds the very shame that makes them worse.

Try This: The Setback Review

When you notice a difficult period beginning, take fifteen minutes to write responses to these four prompts:

What specifically has changed or worsened?

What is happening in my life right now that might be affecting my general anxiety level?

What has worked for me before; which tools, which steps; that I could return to this week?

What would I say to someone I cared about who was going through exactly this?

The fourth prompt is often the most powerful. We are almost always more compassionate to others than to ourselves. Writing the words you would offer a friend, and then reading them back as though they were written for you, can shift the emotional register of a setback from self-condemnation to something more useful: *self-directed kindness.*

Celebrating Progress

If setbacks are the part of the recovery journey that receives the most attention; examined, worried over, and written about at length; progress is often the part that receives the least. Many people with paruresis move past genuine achievements with barely a pause, immediately fixing their gaze on the next challenge, the next limitation, the gap between where they are and where they want to be.

This is not ingratitude. It is a feature of the anxious mind, which is neurologically primed to attend to threat and difficulty far more readily than to safety and success. The brain registers danger in sharp, high-resolution detail. Progress tends to blur into the background unless you deliberately bring it into focus.

Deliberately celebrating progress is not self-indulgence. It is neurologically sound practice. Positive reinforcement, the experience of reward following a successful behaviour, strengthens the neural pathways associated with that behaviour, making it more accessible in the future. When you consciously acknowledge and mark an achievement, you are literally reinforcing the brain circuits that made that achievement possible.

Tracking Achievements

The trigger journal introduced in Chapter 2 has a natural companion: an achievements log. This is a running record not of difficulties, but of successes: every situation navigated, every step on your hierarchy completed, every moment where anxiety was present and you moved forward anyway.

Entries do not need to be dramatic. In fact, the most important entries are often the smallest ones; because small, consistent steps are the actual architecture of recovery, and they deserve to be seen.

An achievements log entry might look like this:

"Tuesday. Used the restroom at the new coffee shop near work. It was quiet but unfamiliar, I'd have rated it a 5 on my anxiety scale six months ago. Today it was a 2. I didn't even notice until I was washing my hands."

That entry, that unremarkable Tuesday morning, represents months of neurological rewiring. It deserves to be written down. It deserves to be read back on harder days, when the mountain path has narrowed and the view has closed in, as evidence of what is genuinely, verifiably true: that you have changed, that progress has happened, that the work is working.

Try This: The Weekly Review

Set aside ten minutes at the end of each week, Sunday evening works well for many people, to review the week specifically for progress. Ask *yourself:*

Was there a situation this week that I handled better than I would have three months ago?

Was there a moment where I used one of my tools and it helped, even partially?

Was there something I did this week, however small, that I wouldn't have been willing to attempt a year ago?

Write at least one genuine answer to at least one of these questions every week. Over months, these entries accumulate into something powerful: *a personal, evidence-based counter-narrative to the story anxiety tells about you.*

Rewards and Reinforcement

Beyond the internal work of acknowledgment, deliberate external rewards have a meaningful role in sustaining motivation, particularly during the sustained, incremental effort that exposure work requires.

The key principle of effective reward is that it should be specific, timely, and proportionate. A reward given immediately after a completed exposure step reinforces that specific behaviour far more powerfully than a vague promise of future reward when the whole hierarchy is complete. The brain learns in the present tense.

Rewards do not need to be elaborate or expensive. They need to be things that genuinely matter to you; ***a favourite meal, a film you have been looking forward to, an hour of unhurried reading, a walk somewhere beautiful, a purchase you have been considering.*** What matters is the deliberate linking of the achievement with something pleasant, creating a positive association that the brain will remember.

Some people find it helpful to establish a milestone reward system at the outset, identifying specific rewards attached to specific hierarchy steps. Completing the first three rungs might earn a small reward. Reaching the midpoint might earn a more significant one. Completing the full hierarchy might earn something genuinely celebratory.

Written in advance and kept somewhere visible, this system serves a dual purpose: ***it provides motivational structure during the work, and it makes concrete, from the beginning, the expectation that success is coming.***

A Word of Encouragement

You have already come further than you may realise. The fact that you are reading this chapter; that you have stayed with this book through six chapters of honest, sometimes difficult, material; is itself evidence of something important: that you have not given up on yourself. That the part of you that wants freedom is stronger than the part that would rather stay safe by staying small.

On the days when progress feels invisible, when a setback has shaken your confidence, when the mountain path has doubled back on itself and you cannot see where you are going, please return to this page. Read these words.

Remember that the path has not disappeared. It is simply winding. And you are still on it.

Questions for Consideration

Take some quiet time to reflect on the following before moving forward:

How have I typically responded to setbacks in the past, in this area or in other areas of my life? Has that response served me? What might a different response look like?

Looking back over the past weeks or months of working with this material, what is one genuine change, however small, that I can honestly identify? Have I given that change the acknowledgment it deserves?

What would a meaningful milestone reward look like for me, something specific that I could give myself when I complete the first three steps of my exposure hierarchy?

Is there a particular context; a type of stress, a life circumstance, a pattern of disrupted sleep or poor self-care; that reliably raises my overall anxiety and therefore my vulnerability to setbacks? What could I do to protect that area of my life more consistently?

CHAPTER 8: LONG-TERM CONFIDENCE AND EMPOWERMENT

This Is Not the End of the Journey; It Is the Beginning of a Different One

There is a particular moment that many people in recovery from paruresis describe, usually some months into the work, when something quietly shifts. It is not always dramatic. Sometimes it is as simple as arriving at a busy venue, walking to the restroom, and realizing; only afterward, on the way back to your seat; that you did not plan it, did not dread it in advance, did not emerge feeling relieved so much as simply... unremarkable. Ordinary. Free.

That ordinariness is the destination. Not the absence of all anxiety forever, that is not a realistic or even necessary goal. But a life in which paruresis occupies so little of your attention, planning, and energy that you can direct those resources toward the things that actually matter to you. **Relationships. Work. Travel. Adventure. Presence. The texture of an ordinary Tuesday, unmanaged and unguarded.**

That life is available to you. This final chapter is about how to build it, and how to sustain it long after you close this book.

Incorporating Skills into Daily Life

Recovery from paruresis does not end when your exposure hierarchy is complete. It transitions, from an active, effortful process of change into a more sustainable practice of maintenance, integration, and continued gentle expansion. The skills you have developed through this book are not temporary scaffolding to be dismantled once the building is standing. They are structuralm and they work best when they become simply part of how you live.

The greatest risk in the later stages of recovery is not relapse through dramatic failure. It is gradual drift; the slow, barely perceptible withdrawal from the practices that have supported your progress, until one day you realise that the breathing exercises have not been practiced in weeks, the achievements log has gone untouched for months, and a few situations that were once comfortably manageable have quietly become difficult again.

Drift is not a character flaw. It is an entirely natural feature of the post-recovery period, when the urgency that drove initial effort has softened, and the practices that once felt urgently necessary begin to feel optional. Managing drift requires building the skills of recovery into the structure of daily life, not as a burden, but as a genuine investment in the freedom you have worked to create.

Daily maintenance practices need not be time-consuming. Research on habit formation and anxiety maintenance consistently shows that brief, consistent practice is more protective than occasional intensive effort. Consider which of the following you might reasonably sustain as background rhythms of daily life:

Five minutes of diaphragmatic breathing each morning before the day begins, not as a crisis intervention, but as a daily calibration of your nervous system's baseline.

A brief weekly review of your achievements log, noting any progress and any situations that felt surprisingly manageable.

Occasional intentional use of restrooms that are slightly outside your comfort zone, not as formal exposure sessions, but as casual maintenance of the neural pathways that tolerate mild challenge without alarm.

These practices, woven into the fabric of an ordinary week, do not feel like therapy. They feel like self-care, because that is precisely what they are.

Try This: Your Maintenance Plan

Write a brief, honest document, it need be no longer than half a page, that answers the following:

Which two or three practices from this book have made the most meaningful difference to my experience of paruresis?

How could I realistically incorporate each of these into a normal week, without making my recovery a second full-time job?

What is my early warning signal, the first sign that tells me my general anxiety is rising or my maintenance practice is slipping, and what will I do when I notice it?

Keep this document somewhere accessible. Review it every few months. Update it as your life changes, because it will, and your maintenance plan should evolve with it.

Adapting to New Challenges

Life does not stay still during recovery, and recovery does not insulate you from the new situations that life reliably generates. *A new job with different restroom arrangements. A relationship that involves more travel. A health challenge that requires medical procedures. A change in living situation.* Each of these can present novel anxiety-provoking contexts that your current hierarchy did not specifically address, and that is not a problem. It is an opportunity to apply what you have learned to fresh terrain.

The skills developed through paruresis work; tolerance of discomfort, graduated approach to feared situations, cognitive flexibility, physiological regulation; are not condition-specific. They are general capabilities that transfer to new challenges with surprising effectiveness.

People who have worked seriously through an exposure hierarchy for paruresis frequently find themselves better equipped to handle other anxiety-provoking situations in their lives: *difficult conversations, performance anxiety, new social contexts*. The paruresis work, it turns out, was also training for something larger.

Amara, 36, had worked through her paruresis hierarchy over eighteen months and reached a point where she could use public restrooms in most situations with mild, manageable anxiety. When she was offered a role that involved international travel, something she had avoided for a decade, she was frightened. The airports, the unfamiliar restrooms, the long flights with pressured timing: all of it loomed.

But she approached it exactly as she had approached her hierarchy. She identified the specific anxiety-provoking elements. She rated them. She began with the least challenging, a short domestic flight, and built from there. Four months later, she flew to Japan for two weeks. *"I won't pretend it was effortless,"* she said. *"But I knew exactly what to do. I had done it before."*

When new challenges arise, trust the process you know. Build a mini-hierarchy if helpful. Return to your breathing and cognitive tools. Reach for your support network. You are not starting from the beginning; you are applying an established skill set to new material. That is a fundamentally different proposition from where you began.

New challenges are not evidence that your recovery was incomplete. They are evidence that your life is expanding, that you are moving into territory that paruresis once kept you from entering.

The anxiety you feel in new situations is not the same anxiety you felt at the beginning of this journey. It is smaller, more manageable, and met by a person with genuine tools and hard-won experience. You are not who you were when you first opened this book. That matters more than you may yet fully realise.

A common misconception about confidence is that it is the absence of fear, that truly confident people simply do not feel anxious in situations where others do. This misconception is particularly damaging in the context of paruresis, where the goal can easily become distorted into "*being someone who never feels anxious in restrooms.*" That goal sets a standard no human nervous system can reliably meet, and it measures confidence by the wrong criteria entirely.

Genuine confidence; the durable kind, built through real experience rather than the absence of difficulty; is not the absence of anxiety. It is the knowledge, grounded in lived evidence, that you can manage anxiety when it arises. It is the accumulated memory of situations you have faced and survived. It is the trust, earned through practice, that your toolkit works, that you have resources to draw on when the familiar freeze begins.

This redefinition of confidence is not a consolation prize. It is, in fact, far more robust than the fragile confidence of someone who has never been tested. The person who has never experienced significant anxiety has no knowledge of what they are capable of when tested. You do. You have faced something genuinely difficult, consistently and repeatedly, and you have moved through it. That is not ordinary. That is extraordinary, even if it has come to feel, appropriately, quite ordinary to you.

Did You Know?

Psychological research on post-traumatic growth, positive psychological change that emerges from struggling with highly challenging life circumstances, has documented consistent patterns of increased personal strength, greater appreciation for life, deeper relationships, and expanded sense of possibility in people who have worked through sustained adversity.

Many people who recover from significant anxiety disorders, including paruresis, describe not simply returning to who they were before, but becoming someone more capable, more compassionate, and more resilient than they had previously been. The struggle, it turns out, was also a teacher.

Inspiring Others

You did not ask to have paruresis. You did not choose the years of management, concealment, and quiet limitation that it has involved. But you are here; at the end of a book about recovery, equipped with knowledge and tools and, very likely, a degree of progress you did not have when you began. And what you carry now has value beyond your own life.

There are, conservatively, millions of people living with paruresis in silence, people at the beginning of the journey you have been walking, who do not yet know that what they are experiencing has a name, a community, or a path forward. Every person who recovers and chooses to speak; to a friend, in an online forum, in a conversation with a healthcare provider; expands the space of possibility for someone who is still silent and still suffering.

You are not obligated to become an advocate. Disclosure is always a personal decision, and choosing to keep your experience private is entirely valid. But if you find, as many people do, that your recovery has given you something you want to share; a sense of what is possible, a reduction in the shame that kept you isolated for so long, a desire to be for someone else the voice that would have helped you; that impulse is worth honouring.

The International Paruresis Association and similar organisations around the world are sustained by people exactly like you: people who found their way through and decided to leave a light on for those still navigating the dark.

Peer support, the kind explored in Chapter 6, is built from recovered voices. The next person who searches desperately online at midnight for any evidence that their experience is real and shared and survivable, they may find your words. And your words may be the thing that changes everything for them, as someone else's words once changed things for you.

<h2 style="text-align:center">Reflection Prompt: Your Recovery Letter</h2>

Write a brief letter, it need never be sent or shown to anyone, to the person you were when paruresis was at its most limiting. Tell them what you know now that they did not know then. Tell them what became possible. Tell them what the work felt like, and what it was worth.

Write it honestly, without minimising the difficulty or performing a happiness you do not feel. Then read it back, slowly, as the person you are now. Notice what it contains. Notice what you have lived through. Notice who you have become.

<h3 style="text-align:center">Questions for Consideration</h3>

As you complete this book and look toward the continuing journey ahead, take time with these final questions:

Looking at my life now compared to when I began this work, what has genuinely changed? Not in ideal terms, but in honest ones. What can I do now that I could not do before? What do I understand about myself that I did not understand before?

What does long-term confidence mean to me, personally, not in terms of paruresis specifically, but in terms of the kind of person I am becoming and the life I am building?

Is there one person, in my life or in an online community, to whom my experience and progress might be genuinely useful? Is there something I could share, however briefly, that might matter to them?

What is one thing I want to do; one experience I want to have, one freedom I want to reclaim; that paruresis has prevented until now? Can I name it clearly, and can I begin to move toward it?

CONCLUSION
When Nature Calls, You Will Be Ready

You came to this book carrying something heavy. Perhaps you had been carrying it for years: **the daily calculations, the mapping of exits, the quiet grief of experiences missed and freedoms foregone**. Perhaps you had never told a single person. Perhaps you had almost convinced yourself that this was simply who you were, that the territory paruresis had claimed was territory permanently lost.

It was not. It never was.

What this book has tried to offer; through science and story, through practical tools and honest reflection, through the voices of composite people whose experiences mirror your own; is a single, fundamental truth: paruresis is not a life sentence. It is a condition with a well-understood mechanism, a clear evidence base for treatment, and a path forward that is genuinely, demonstrably available to people who have lived with it at every level of severity, for every length of time.

The path is not always easy. You have seen that clearly across these eight chapters. It requires the particular courage of showing up repeatedly for something uncomfortable, of meeting setbacks with curiosity rather than despair, of being willing to ask for help and accept support and tell the truth about your experience to people who can hold it with care. That kind of courage is quiet and unsexy and completely, utterly real.

You have also seen; in Oliver and Priya and James and Nina and Amara and Thomas and Diane and Marcus, in all the composite lives woven through these pages; that the work is finite. That hierarchies are completed. That situations which once produced overwhelming anxiety become manageable and then ordinary. That lives genuinely, measurably expand. That the restroom in the airport is eventually just a restroom.

What you do with this book from here is yours to decide. Perhaps you will begin your trigger journal this week, or write your first fear hierarchy, or make an appointment with a therapist, or join an online community. Perhaps you will tell one person, just one, about something you have carried alone for far too long.

Perhaps you will simply sit with what you have read and let it settle, finding the courage to begin when you are ready.

All of these are right. All of these are enough. The only wrong move is to put the book down and return to the silence and the avoidance and the daily management of a life shaped around a fear that does not have to define you.

You picked this book up. Something in you; the part that wants freedom, the part that has not given up, the part that knows there is more available to you than this; made that choice. Trust that part. It has been right all along.

When nature calls, you will be ready.

A Final Word

Recovery is not a destination you arrive at and then possess forever unchanged. It is a practice; an ongoing, evolving relationship with yourself, your nervous system, and the world of situations you are reclaiming. There will be good days and harder ones. There will be moments of quiet triumph and moments of frustration. Through all of them, you are not alone.

The community of people who understand this experience, who have walked this path and left lights on for those coming behind, is real, and it includes you now. You belong to it. You always did.

Welcome.

INDEX

Note: Entries are referenced by chapter (e.g., Ch. 1) and section location. Entries marked (Ex) indicate exercises or practical tools; (CS) indicates composite case studies.

- and fear extinction, Ch. 4

- and social anxiety, Ch. 1

- MBSR effects on, Ch. 3

- role in paruresis, Ch. 1

anticipatory anxiety

- defined, Ch. 1

- frequency relative to in-the-moment anxiety, Ch. 2

- mindfulness as treatment for, Ch. 3

- *See also anxiety*

anxiety

- anticipatory, Ch. 1, Ch. 2, Ch. 3

- as nervous system response, Ch. 1, Ch. 5

- in-the-moment vs. anticipated, Ch. 2

- rating scale (0–10), Ch. 2, Ch. 4

- *See also social anxiety disorder*

anxiety rating scale (SUDS)

- in exposure hierarchy, Ch. 4

- in trigger journal, Ch. 2

- moderate range for effective exposure, Ch. 4

- *See also Subjective Units of Distress Scale (SUDS)*

audience, perceived** See observation, perceived

automatic negative thoughts

- defined, Ch. 3

- identifying, Ch. 3

- *See also cognitive distortions; thought record*

C

careers and employment

- drug testing requirements, Ch. 1, Ch. 6

- impact of paruresis on, Ch. 1

- promotion avoidance (James case study), Ch. 1

case studies See individual names: Amara; Diane; James; Marcus; Nina; Oliver; Priya; Thomas

catastrophic thinking (catastrophising)

- defined, Ch. 3

- in paruresis, Ch. 2, Ch. 3

- reframing, Ch. 3

- *See also cognitive distortions*

CBT See Cognitive Behavioural Therapy (CBT)

classical conditioning

- and paruresis triggers, Ch. 2

- defined, Ch. 2

- *See also triggers*

Clinical Psychology Review (journal), Ch. 7

cognitive appraisal, Ch. 2

Cognitive Behavioural Therapy (CBT)

- Aaron Beck and Albert Ellis, Ch. 3

- automatic negative thoughts, Ch. 3

- cognitive distortions, Ch. 3

- for paruresis, Ch. 3, Ch. 6

- guided/Socratic questioning, Ch. 3

disclosure

- framing the conversation, Ch. 6

- online communities and, Ch. 6

- personal decision, Ch. 6, Ch. 8

- principles for telling someone, Ch. 6

- research on anticipation vs. actual response, Ch. 6

- *See also support networks*

distress rating See anxiety rating scale (SUDS)

drift (post-recovery), Ch. 8

- *See also relapse prevention*

drug testing, Ch. 1, Ch. 6

DSM-5 See Diagnostic and Statistical Manual of Mental Disorders

G

graduated exposure therapy

- basics of, Ch. 4

- evidence base, Ch. 4

- fear hierarchy, Ch. 4

- flooding distinguished from, Ch. 4

- gradual steps rationale, Ch. 4

- in setback recovery, Ch. 7

- moderate anxiety range for, Ch. 4

- practicing safely, Ch. 4

- research (Journal of Anxiety Disorders), Ch. 4

- tracking progress, Ch. 4

- *See also fear hierarchy; fear extinction*

group therapy, Ch. 6

- *See also therapy modalities*

grounding See 5-4-3-2-1 grounding practice

guided questioning See Socratic questioning

guided visualisation See visualisation

H

habit formation, Ch. 8

Hayes, Steven**, Ch. 3

heart rate variability (HRV), Ch. 5

- See also parasympathetic nervous system

hypervigilance See body hypervigilance

I

IPA See International Paruresis Association

International Paruresis Association (IPA)

- peer support groups, Ch. 6

- prevalence statistics, Ch. 1

- website and resources, Ch. 6, Ch. 8

isolation, Introduction, Ch. 1, Ch. 6

- See also emotional consequences of paruresis; shame

J

Jacobson, Edmund**, Ch. 5

James (composite case study) (CS), Ch. 1

Journal of Anxiety Disorders, Ch. 4

Journal of Neurophysiology, Ch. 5

journaling

- achievements log, Ch. 7

- recovery letter (Ex), Ch. 8

- trigger journal, Ch. 2, Ch. 4

- weekly review (Ex), Ch. 7

- See also reflection prompts

Mindfulness-Based Stress Reduction (MBSR)

- amygdala effects, Ch. 3

- developer (Jon Kabat-Zinn), Ch. 3

- evidence base, Ch. 3

- for paruresis, Ch. 3

- origins, Ch. 3

motivation See rewards and reinforcement; setbacks, staying motivated

muscle tension, Ch. 1, Ch. 5

- *See also progressive muscle relaxation*

N

negative thoughts See automatic negative thoughts; cognitive distortions

nervous system

- parasympathetic, Ch. 1, Ch. 5

- sympathetic, Ch. 1, Ch. 2, Ch. 5

- vagus nerve, Ch. 5

- *See also brain; fight-or-flight response*

neural pathways

- building new pathways through exposure, Ch. 4

- visualisation and, Ch. 5

- *See also fear extinction; graduated exposure therapy*

Nina (composite case study) (CS), Ch. 4, Conclusion

noise and silence (as trigger)

- acoustic environment, Ch. 2, Ch. 5

- background noise as aid, Ch. 5

- white noise apps, Ch. 5

- *See also privacy strategies; triggers, environmental*

normalising setbacks **See setbacks**, normalising

O

observation, perceived**

- as core mechanism, Ch. 5

- observer effect research, Ch. 5

- *See also privacy strategies; triggers, psychological*

Oliver (composite case study) (CS), Ch. 7, Conclusion

online communities, Ch. 6, Ch. 8

- *See also peer support groups*

P

parasympathetic nervous system

- and urination, Ch. 1

- breathing and, Ch. 5

- heart rate variability (HRV), Ch. 5

- vagus nerve, Ch. 5

- *See also nervous system*

paruresis

- as social anxiety disorder, Ch. 1

- causes and mechanisms, Ch. 1

- defined and explained, Ch. 1

- DSM-5 recognition, Ch. 1

- emotional consequences, Ch. 1

W

weekly review (Ex), Ch. 7

white noise See noise and silence (as trigger); privacy strategies

witnessed drug testing See drug testing

Z

zero-to-ten anxiety scale See anxiety rating scale (SUDS)

www.ingramcontent.com/pod-product-compliance
Lightning Source LLC
Chambersburg PA
CBHW050803250726

48653CB00006B/2054